"Radiant Expectations: Embracing Style during Pregnancy"

Sharon Shante

Every woman who is pregnant and wants to maintain
a stylish look during pregnancy.

CONTENTS

INTRODUCTION

Pregnancy is a transformative journey with challenges, including finding comfortable and fashionable clothing. As your body changes and grows, finding clothing that fits well and makes you feel confident and beautiful can be challenging. However, it is essential to prioritise comfort and style during this time to help you feel good, both physically and emotionally.

The good news is that there are many ways to dress fashionably during pregnancy, no matter your style or body type. With some knowledge and creativity, you can embrace your changing body and enjoy the journey in style.

This book, "Radiant Expectations: Embracing Style during Pregnancy, is a guide to dressing for pregnancy, offering practical tips and advice on how to look and feel your best throughout this beautiful journey.

In this book, you will learn about the different stages of pregnancy and how your body changes during each trimester. You will discover the best types of clothing to wear at each stage and how to mix and match different pieces to create stylish and comfortable outfits. You will also learn about accessorising during pregnancy and how to use accessories to draw attention to your best features and away from areas you may be self-conscious about.

However, this book is not just about fashion but also about embracing your changing body and enjoying the pregnancy journey. You will learn about the importance of self-care during pregnancy and how to prioritise your mental and emotional well-being.

Most importantly, this book empowers you to feel confident and beautiful during this transformative journey. You will learn to embrace your changing body and appreciate all the fantastic things it is doing to create a new life. Whether you are a first-time mother or a seasoned pro, this book has something for everyone who wants to look and feel their best during pregnancy.

So, whether you are a fashionista or just looking for practical tips on dressing for pregnancy, "Pregnant and Stylish" is the ultimate guide to help you look and feel your best during this beautiful journey. Let us dive in, discover the world of pregnancy fashion and style, and embrace the journey with confidence.

PREFACE

Pregnancy is a truly beautiful phase in a woman's life, filled with both joys and challenges. However, it can be especially difficult to dress up during this time due to the numerous changes that the body undergoes. That's why I wrote this guidebook to help all expecting mothers look and feel their best. From choosing the right maternity wear to accessorizing, this book has everything you need to know to embrace your style and feel confident during this journey of motherhood. My hope is that this book inspires you to celebrate the beauty of this phase in your life and enjoy every moment.

PROLOGUE

Pregnancy is a phase in a woman's life, and it is natural to want to look and feel our best during this time. However, finding the right clothes that fit and flatter our changing bodies can be daunting. The fashion industry's limited options for maternity wear often make it challenging to stay stylish and confident.

"Pregnant and Stylish," is a book to help you make the most of your wardrobe during pregnancy. Whether you are a first-time mom or a seasoned pro, this book will provide the tools and inspiration to embrace your unique style and feel confident every step of the way.

We will explore how to dress for your body type, mix

and match your existing clothes, and choose the right accessories to enhance your look. You will learn how to stay comfortable without compromising style and discover the best places to shop for maternity wear.

With "Pregnant and Stylish," you will have everything you need to look and feel your best during this beautiful time.

CHAPTER 1

PREGNANCY AND FASHION

Pregnancy is a beautiful journey filled with excitement, anticipation, and joy. As an expecting mother, you are preparing to bring a new life into the world and embark on a journey of self-discovery and personal growth. One aspect of this journey that many women struggle with is fashion. With a rapidly changing body and a limited selection of clothing, it can be challenging to feel stylish and confident during pregnancy. However, with some knowledge and creativity, you can embrace your changing body and enjoy the pregnancy journey in style.

The first step in dressing for pregnancy is understanding your body and how it changes each trimester. You may not notice many physical changes during the first trimester, but choosing comfortable and accommodating clothing is still important. Look for loose-fitting tops and dresses that accommodate any bloating or changes in breast size. You may also want to invest in a comfortable pair of leggings or stretchy pants that can grow with you throughout your pregnancy.

As you move into the second trimester, you will likely notice more significant changes in your body. Your belly will start to grow, and you may find that your regular clothing no longer fits comfortably. This is the time to start investing in maternity wear. Maternity wear is designed to accommodate a growing belly and provide comfort and support where you need it most. Look for clothing made from stretchy, breathable fabrics and adjustable waistbands or panels that can grow with you.

During the third trimester, your belly will be much larger, and you will need to focus on clothing that provides support and comfort while still looking fashionable. Maxi dresses, flowy tops, and loose-fitting pants are all great options for this stage of pregnancy. You may also want to invest in a few key pieces, such as a comfortable pair of maternity jeans or a supportive belly band, to help you feel confident and comfortable throughout your pregnancy.

Regarding accessorising during pregnancy, there are a few things to remember. First, focus on accessories that add comfort and functionality to your outfits. Comfortable shoes with good support are essential during pregnancy, especially as your body weight shifts and your centre of gravity changes. Look for shoes with a low heel or no heel at all, and make sure they fit well and provide ample support. You may also want to invest in a supportive bra that can accommodate changes in breast size and provide the help you need.

During pregnancy, accessories can create a focal point and draw attention away from self-conscious areas. For example, if you feel self-conscious about your growing belly, try wearing a statement necklace or bold earrings that draw attention to your face instead.

To conclude, the journey of pregnancy and fashion is both exciting and challenging. Nevertheless, armed with some knowledge and creativity, you can embrace your changing body and enjoy the journey in style. Remember to choose clothing that is comfortable and accommodating, invest in maternity wear that provides the necessary support and comfort, and focus on accessories that add functionality while highlighting your best features.

CHAPTER 2

COMFORT AND FASHION

Pregnancy is an incredible journey that comes with its own set of unique challenges. One of the biggest challenges is finding comfortable clothes that still look fashionable. As your body changes and grows, finding clothing that fits properly and feels comfortable can be complex. However, it is essential to prioritise comfort during this time, as it can significantly impact your overall well-being.

Comfortable clothing is about feeling good physically, mentally, and emotionally. When you are comfortable in your clothes, you are more likely to feel confident, positive, and happy. Conversely, when you are uncomfortable, it can make you feel self-conscious and unhappy. This is why choosing clothing that makes you feel good from the inside out is important.

During pregnancy, the body constantly changes and finding clothing that accommodates those changes can be challenging. However, there are a few key things to keep in mind when it comes to choosing comfortable clothing that still looks fashionable.

First and foremost, prioritise fabrics that are soft, stretchy, and breathable. Your body temperature can fluctuate during pregnancy, and you may experience hot flashes or night sweats. Choosing breathable fabrics such as cotton, bamboo, or linen can help keep you cool and comfortable. Additionally, stretchy materials such as spandex or elastane can help accommodate a growing belly and provide support where you need it most.

Another essential factor to consider is fit. When

choosing clothing during pregnancy, selecting items that fit correctly without being too tight or constricting is necessary. Look for apparel specifically for pregnancy, as these items will be designed to accommodate a growing belly and provide the right amount of support. Maternity leggings, for example, often feature a wide, stretchy waistband that can be worn over or under your belly, providing support and comfort throughout the day.

Regarding tops and dresses, look for flowy and loose-fitting items. These garments can provide ample room for a growing belly while still looking fashionable. Empire waist tops and dresses are also great options, as they give a defined waistline while allowing plenty of room in the belly area.

It is also important to consider the length of your clothing when choosing items during pregnancy. Longer tops and tunics can be more comfortable and flattering than shorter, tighter shirts. Additionally, longer dresses and skirts can provide ample coverage while allowing movement and comfort.

When it comes to footwear, prioritise comfort and support over fashion. During pregnancy, your centre of gravity shifts, and you may experience back pain or foot swelling. Choosing shoes with a low heel or no heel can help alleviate some of this discomfort. Look for shoes designed for comfort and support, such as athletic shoes or sandals with arch support.

Finally, do not be afraid to accessorise! Accessories can add a pop of style to any outfit and do not have to be uncomfortable. Scarves, hats, and jewellery are all great options for adding a touch of class to your pregnancy wardrobe without sacrificing comfort.

Choosing fashionable clothes for pregnancy is essential

for your overall well-being. By prioritising soft, stretchy, and breathable fabrics, choosing the right fit, and selecting footwear that prioritises comfort and support, you can create a pregnancy wardrobe that makes you feel confident, comfortable, and stylish.

*Pregnancy is a unique and beautiful journey;
your clothing should reflect that!*

CHAPTER 3

MATERNITY WEARS

Maternity wear is a type of clothing specifically designed for pregnant women. The primary purpose of maternity wear is to provide comfort and support to the expecting mother's changing body while also allowing her to look stylish.

Maternity wear is designed to fit and flatter your changing body, providing comfort and support while looking fashionable. Dressing stylishly during pregnancy is not impossible. With the proper knowledge and tips, you can choose maternity wear that is both comfortable and fashionable. Invest in some essential pieces, choose the right fit, experiment with colours and patterns, accessorise, choose comfortable shoes, and embrace your style.

When it comes to the basics of maternity wear, there are a few key pieces that every pregnant woman should consider investing in.

BASICS OF MATERNITY WEAR

Maternity jeans or pants - Maternity pants have a stretchy waistband that can be adjusted as your belly grows, providing comfort and support.

Maternity tops are available in various styles, from loose blouses to snug t-shirts. Selecting comfortable tops that can easily accommodate your expanding belly is essential. Opt for tops made from soft, stretchable materials that flexibly adjust to your body changes during pregnancy.

Maternity dresses - Dresses are an excellent option for pregnant women as they are comfortable, easy to wear, and can be dressed up or down. Look for breathable fabrics with a loose-fitting silhouette that will grow with your belly.

Maternity bras - Invest in a supportive bra with adjustable straps and a wide band to accommodate breast changes during pregnancy.

Belly band - A belly band is a flexible band designed to fit over your belly, offering support and comfort. It can be worn over or under your clothes and is particularly helpful for women who want to continue wearing their regular pants throughout their pregnancy.

When you go out to buy maternity clothes, selecting garments that are comfortable, practical, and trendy is crucial. Search for items that can expand with you throughout your pregnancy and can be combined and matched to create various outfits. You can feel confident and at ease on your pregnancy journey with the appropriate pieces in your closet.

1. INVEST IN BASICS

To build a fashionable maternity wardrobe, the first step is to purchase some essential pieces that can be combined in different ways to create a variety of outfits. Some examples of these pieces include comfortable maternity jeans, leggings, basic tees and tanks, and a versatile dress. It is important to choose comfortable pieces made from breathable fabrics designed to fit and flatter your changing body.

2. CHOOSE THE RIGHT FIT

Proper fit is crucial when it comes to maternity wear. Tight clothes can be uncomfortable and restrict movement, while loose ones can be unflattering. The best option is to look for clothes specifically designed to fit and flatter your changing body, with ample space for your growing belly. Maternity clothes with adjustable waistbands or panels can be an excellent choice as they can be modified to fit your body as it changes.

3. EXPERIMENT WITH COLOURS AND PATTERNS

Maternity wear does not have to be dull or unexciting. You can be creative with various colours and patterns to add some interest to your wardrobe. Opt for bold colours or patterns that brighten your outfit or a classic look with neutral colours. However, choosing colours and patterns that flatter your skin tone and body shape is important.

4. ACCESSORIZE

Adding accessories to your maternity outfits can be a simple and affordable way to enhance your style and express your personality. Scarves, hats, jewellery, and bags are all great options that elevate your look and make you feel confident. Opt for accessories that complement your outfits and make you feel comfortable.

5. SHOES

During pregnancy, your feet might go through a lot of stress and discomfort. Therefore, choosing shoes that provide comfort, support, and cushioning is crucial. High heels should be avoided as they can put excessive pressure on your feet. Opt for shoes with a low or no heel, such as sneakers, flats, and sandals with good arch support.

6. EMBRACE YOUR STYLE

During pregnancy, it is essential to remember that your style can remain unchanged while wearing maternity clothes. Whether you prefer a classic, bohemian, or trendy style, options are available to match your taste. Do not be afraid to experiment and have fun with different outfits and looks.

Create a maternity wardrobe that makes you feel confident, beautiful and stylish throughout your pregnancy journey.

CHAPTER 4

DRESSING FOR DIFFERENT OCCASIONS

Dressing for different occasions during pregnancy can be challenging, whether you are headed to the office or a formal event. Pregnancy is a beautiful and exciting journey but comes with unique challenges, including finding the perfect outfit for different occasions. When dealing with a rapidly changing body and limited clothing options, creating a stylish and comfortable wardrobe that works for any event can seem daunting. However, you can achieve this goal with some knowledge and creativity.

CASUAL OUTFIT IDEAS

Casual outfits are an excellent choice for daily wear, whether running errands, meeting friends for lunch, or just lounging at home. Comfort is paramount during pregnancy, and numerous casual outfit options can keep you both comfy and stylish.

One easy and comfortable outfit idea is to pair a loose-fitting tunic top with leggings or stretchy pants. This outfit is perfect for early pregnancy when you may not yet be showing up or later when you want to flaunt your bump. For a comfortable and casual look, you can also opt for a simple t-shirt dress paired with sneakers.

For a more sophisticated casual look, try layering pieces together. A long cardigan paired with a T-shirt and jeans can create a chic and cosy look. Adding a scarf or statement necklace can elevate the outfit even more.

WORK OUTFIT IDEAS

Dressing for work while pregnant can be challenging, especially if there is a specific dress code. However, many comfortable and professional outfit options can make you look polished and put together.

One classic work outfit idea is to pair a well-tailored blazer with a comfortable dress or skirt. It is best to look for pieces with some stretch to accommodate your growing belly. Another option is to choose a wrap dress that can be adjusted to fit your stomach as it grows.

A comfortable blouse paired with dress pants or a pencil skirt can be a great choice for expecting mothers. It's important to choose tops made from breathable fabrics like cotton or silk that have some stretch to accommodate your growing bump. Adding a belt above your bump can help define your waist and give a more polished look to your outfit.

FORMAL OUTFIT IDEAS

Dressing up for formal occasions during pregnancy can be pretty challenging, but it is still possible to look stunning and feel comfortable. The key to nailing your look is choosing dresses specifically designed for pregnant women, offering the necessary support and comfort.

An elegant option is a floor-length gown with a fitted top and a flowing skirt. This style can elongate your body and provide a flattering silhouette. Look for dresses with a defined waistline or empire waist to create a more defined shape.

Another great choice is a midi or maxi dress with a wrap-style top. This style can provide comfort and elegance and is perfect for formal events such as weddings.

Regardless of the occasion, the key to dressing up for pregnancy is selecting comfortable, flattering clothing that reflects your style. Do not be afraid to experiment with different types and accessories. Remember to prioritise your comfort and well-being. With these tips, you can create a stylish and comfortable wardrobe for any occasion during your pregnancy.

CHAPTER 5

STAYING ACTIVE AND STYLISH

Staying active during pregnancy is essential for the health of the mother and the baby. However, finding comfortable and stylish clothing that accommodates the changes in a woman's body during pregnancy can be challenging. In this chapter, we will explore the world of activewear for pregnancy and provide tips on choosing the right pieces for your needs.

Pregnancy changes a woman's body significantly, making it crucial to dress appropriately and comfortably, especially when engaging in physical activities. Activewear designed for pregnancy has gained popularity recently, as it provides support, comfort, and flexibility to pregnant women engaging in physical activities. This chapter will discuss some critical factors when choosing activewear for pregnancy.

The most crucial factor to consider when selecting activewear for pregnancy is comfort. Comfort should be the top priority. During pregnancy, the body undergoes significant changes, and choosing clothing that accommodates these changes is essential. The activewear should be made of soft, breathable fabric that is gentle on the skin. It should also be stretchy and flexible to allow freedom of movement. The clothing should fit well to avoid any discomfort or irritation. Staying active during pregnancy is crucial for your and your baby's health. However, finding comfortable and fashionable activewear can be challenging.

Pregnancy changes a woman's body significantly, so it is essential to dress appropriately and comfortably, particularly when engaging in physical activities.

Activewear for pregnancy is a relatively new clothing category that has gained popularity. It is designed to offer comfort, support, and flexibility to pregnant women who engage in physical activities.

The first and most crucial factor to consider is comfort. When choosing activewear, the clothing should be form-fitting for high-intensity activities such as running or aerobics pregnancy, and it is necessary to select clothing that accommodates these changes. Soft, breathable fabric that is gentle on the skin is ideal. The activewear should also be stretchy and flexible to allow freedom of movement. It should fit well to avoid any discomfort or irritation.

When choosing suitable active wear during pregnancy, support is a crucial factor that should not be overlooked. Expecting mothers require adequate support, especially when engaging in physical activities. The ideal activewear should support the growing belly, breasts, and back and include a supportive bra that can accommodate changes in breast size. The clothing should also feature a belly band that supports the growing belly and reduces the risk of back pain. Overall, the clothing should support the entire body, reducing the risk of injuries during physical activities.

When selecting suitable activewear during pregnancy, it is crucial to consider the level of physical activity. Pregnant women participate in various physical activities, and the activewear should match the activity level. Loose-fitting clothes such as leggings and tank tops are suitable for low-intensity activities like yoga, Pilates, and stretching. The clothing should be form-fitting for high-intensity activities such as running or aerobics to minimise movement and reduce the risk of injury.

Another crucial factor to consider is the stage of pregnancy. The clothing should be designed to accommodate the changes in the body during each trimester. During the first trimester, activewear should be loose-fitting to accommodate any bloating or changes in breast size. The clothing should support the growing belly and breasts in the second and third trimesters. The belly band should be made of stretchy fabric that can accommodate the growth of the stomach.

Lastly, it is essential to consider style. Activewear for pregnancy should not compromise style. The clothing should be stylish, making the pregnant woman feel confident and beautiful. The activewear should be available in various colours and designs, allowing the pregnant woman to express her style.

Active wear for pregnancy is an essential clothing category for pregnant women who engage in physical activities. When choosing active wear for pregnancy, it is important to consider comfort, support, activity level, stage of pregnancy, and style. The clothing should be made of soft and breathable fabric that is gentle on the skin. It should provide support to the growing belly, breasts, and back.

The clothing should match the activity level and stage of pregnancy. Lastly, the dress should be fashionable, making the pregnant woman feel confident and beautiful. With these factors in mind, pregnant women can choose suitable activewear that matches their pregnancy journey and allows them to engage in physical activities comfortably and confidently.

CHAPTER 6

THE JOY OF ACCESSORIES

ccessories are essential for any outfit, especially for pregnant women. They help to make them look fashionable, stylish, and confident. With the right accessories, a pregnant woman can easily divert attention from areas she may be self-conscious about, add personality to her outfit, and create a polished, put-together look that makes her feel comfortable and confident.

During pregnancy, accessories can be used to add colour or a statement piece to an otherwise plain outfit. For instance, if you wear a simple black or white dress, you can add a statement necklace or a pair of bold earrings to add colour and personality to the outfit, showcasing your style and adding flair to your wardrobe.

In addition, accessories can help pregnant women look fashionable by drawing attention away from changing or growing areas such as the belly. Using scarves, hats, or statement jewellery can divert attention away from your midsection and towards your face or neck, making you feel more comfortable and confident in your outfit.

Furthermore, accessories can help balance a pregnant woman's silhouette and create a more flattering overall look. Wearing a loose-fitting top or dress with a belt can define your waistline and create a more hourglass shape, boosting your confidence and making you feel comfortable.

During pregnancy, choosing comfortable shoes that provide good support is essential. This is because your body weight is shifting, and your centre of gravity is changing. However, you do not have to compromise on style for comfort. Wear stylish, comfortable shoes like loafers, ballet flats, or low-heeled boots. You can even choose shoes with fun prints or bold colours to add personality to your outfit.

Additionally, accessories can help create a cohesive overall look, tying your outfit together. You can choose accessories that match your outfit's colour or style, such as a necklace that complements the print on your dress or a scarf that matches your shoes' colour. This creates a polished, put-together look, making you feel confident, fashionable, and ready to take on the day.

Fashion accessories can add personality and style to your pregnancy wardrobe.

HERE ARE SOME TIPS ON HOW

TO USE FASHION ACCESSORIES AS A PREGNANT WOMAN:

1. **Scarves**

Scarves are versatile accessories that can add a bold statement piece or a delicate one; jewellery significantly impacts add layers or tie it around your neck for a pop of colour. During pregnancy, scarves can be a stylish and practical accessory that comes in handy. They can add a pop of colour or texture to your outfit while also providing comfort and warmth. One way to wear a scarf during pregnancy is to use it as a belt. You can wrap it around your waist, tie a knot or bow, and adjust it as needed. This can accentuate your growing belly while adding a stylish touch to your outfit.

Another way to wear a scarf is as a headband or hair accessory. With hair becoming more challenging to manage during pregnancy, the scarf can be a stylish and practical solution. You can wrap it around your head, tie it in a knot, or bow at the top and tuck in any loose ends. Scarves can also be used as a shawl or wrap, providing warmth and comfort during cooler weather. You drape the scarf over your shoulders and adjust it as needed or wrap it around your body for added warmth.

In addition to these ideas, scarves can be worn as a statement piece, adding a pop of colour or texture to your outfit. You can drape the scarf around your neck or shoulders or tie it in a knot for a more structured look. In summary, scarves are a versatile and practical accessory during pregnancy. By experimenting with different styles and techniques, you can add a fashionable touch to your outfit while staying comfortable and cosy.

2. Jewellery

Jewellery is an indispensable fashion accessory that enhances any outfit and makes a pregnant woman look fashionable. It adds elegance, sophistication, or playfulness to an outfit and helps to create a personal style statement. Whether a bold statement piece or a delicate one, jewellery significantly impacts a woman's overall look and style.

Firstly, jewellery adds glamour and elegance to an outfit. A statement necklace or chandelier earrings can transform a simple outfit into a chic look. It creates a focal point and draws attention to a specific feature, such as the neckline or wrists, to create a balanced and polished look.

Secondly, jewellery expresses personal style and adds a unique touch to an outfit. From delicate and understated pieces to bold and dramatic statement pieces, jewellery reflects a woman's personality and individuality. It adds colour or texture to an outfit and creates a visually exciting look.

Thirdly, jewellery complements an outfit and creates a cohesive look. Matching jewellery, such as a necklace or bracelet, to the colour or style of an outfit ties the look together and creates a polished and cohesive appearance. It also adds contrast and creates an interesting visual effect.

Lastly, jewellery creates a playful and fun look. Mixing and matching different jewellery pieces, such as stacking bracelets or layering necklaces, creates a trendy and playful look perfect for casual occasions. Unique and eclectic pieces of jewellery add a bohemian or vintage-inspired look.

In conclusion, jewellery is a fashion accessory that adds glamour and personal style to complement an outfit and create a look that is uniquely her own. It adds glamour and personal style and complements an outfit to create a polished and fashionable look that is uniquely hers.

3. Belts

Belts are a versatile accessory that can add style and definition to any outfit. For pregnant women, belts can be a great way to create a waistline and accentuate the baby bump. Choosing the correct type of belt and wearing it comfortably and safely during pregnancy is essential.

The first step in using belts as an accessory during pregnancy is to choose the right belt type. Wide belts that sit low on the hips are a good option, as they can help create a defined waistline without putting pressure on the baby bump. Stretchy belts made from elastic materials, such as spandex or elastane, can also be a great choice, as they can stretch to accommodate a growing belly.

During pregnancy, it is essential to wear a belt comfortably and safely. Avoid wearing the belt too tight or high on the belly, as this can cause discomfort and put pressure on the uterus. Instead, wear the belt under the belly or low on the hips to alleviate unnecessary stress.

Belts can be a great accessory to elevate pregnancy outfits, such as dresses, tunics, tops, or leggings. They can add a pop of colour or texture or help create a more defined silhouette. For example, wearing a wide belt over a loose-fitting maxi dress can accentuate the waistline and create shape.

Belts can serve as a fantastic accessory for expectant mothers who desire to elevate the style and contour of their ensembles. Choosing a comfortable and safe belt during pregnancy makes expecting mothers feel confident and fashionable.

4. Hats

Hats are a versatile accessory that can add a touch

of style to any outfit, including pregnancy wear. The perfect hat can elevate your look and provide practical benefits such as protection from the sun or cold weather. Hats can be a great fashion accessory during pregnancy, offering style and practicality. By incorporating hats into your pregnancy outfits, you can feel confident and fashionable throughout your pregnancy journey.

When choosing the right hat during pregnancy, remember a few things. Firstly, consider the size and shape of your head. As your body changes during pregnancy, your head size may also increase. Therefore, try on hats before purchasing them to ensure a comfortable fit.

When selecting a hat, it is essential to consider its purpose. For instance, if the hat is for protection from the sun or warmth during colder months, different types of hats, such as wide-brimmed sun hats or cosy beanies, may be needed.

Additionally, the style of the hat is another crucial factor to consider. A wide range of hat styles is available, from classic fedoras to trendy bucket hats. Selecting a style that aligns with personal taste and works well with one's pregnancy wardrobe is crucial.

One way to incorporate hats into the pregnancy wardrobe is by choosing hats that match the outfit. For instance, a wide-brimmed sun hat can add a touch of elegance and protect the face from the sun when paired with a flowy maxi dress. A baseball cap or beanie can add a casual touch to the outfit for a more laid-back look. Hats can also add a pop of colour to a neutral or monochromatic outfit, adding interest and personality to the overall look.

5. Bags

The selection of a bag during pregnancy is a crucial decision that requires attention to various factors, including size, shape, functionality, and fashion. As a practical item, the bag should offer enough room to carry essential items, such as water bottles, snacks, and extra clothes.

However, it is equally important to choose a bag that complements the outfit and enhances the style of the pregnant woman. In this regard, tote bags emerge as an excellent option due to their ample space and versatility. They are available in various materials, such as canvas or leather, and can be dressed up or down, making them a practical and stylish choice for everyday use.

Pregnant women can choose tote bags to meet their functional and fashionable needs while carrying essential items. Another great option is backpacks. They distribute weight evenly across the back, reducing strain on the shoulders and neck. Backpacks are available in various materials, including leather and nylon, and can be dressed up or down for a functional and fashionable look.

Crossbody bags have become popular for individuals who value convenience and mobility. These bags are designed to be worn across the body or over the shoulder, providing a practical and stylish option for everyday use. Available in various materials, such as leather or nylon, crossbody bags can be dressed up or down to match any outfit, making them a versatile accessory in contemporary, stylish and functional bag right bag during pregnancy, the choice can be perplexing.

Choosing a stylish and functional bag is crucial, allowing the expecting mother to carry all the essentials while still looking chic. There are two primary options to consider: clutch bags and shoulder bags.

Clutch bags are an ideal choice for special occasions. They come in various materials, such as leather and satin, and offer a sophisticated look. On the other hand, shoulder bags are more versatile and can be dressed up or down. They come in materials like leather or suede and are perfect for everyday use. These bags can be worn on the shoulder or across the body, providing pregnant women flexibility and ease of use.

It is important to choose bags that offer practicality and style. As a pregnant woman, having a bag that can hold all the essentials, such as water bottles, snacks, and extra clothing, is essential while still looking fashionable. Accessories like bags should be comfortable and functional, making the mother-to-be feel confident. With a bit of creativity, these bags can create a stylish and comfortable pregnancy wardrobe, allowing expecting mothers to look and feel their best.

CHAPTER 7

EMBRACING YOUR STYLE

Pregnant women should embrace their personal style when it comes to dressing during pregnancy. Doing so can significantly impact their overall well-being by making them feel more comfortable, confident, and empowered throughout their pregnancy journey.

Embracing one's style during pregnancy can help women feel more comfortable in their skin. Pregnancy can be a time of self-doubt and insecurity, and with so many changes happening in the body, it can be challenging to feel confident about one's appearance. However, embracing their style makes women feel more positive about their appearance, boosting their overall well-being.

Furthermore, embracing one's style during pregnancy can make women feel more empowered and in control. Pregnancy can be an uncertain time, and it can be challenging to feel like one has control over their body and life. By embracing their style, women can take control of their appearance and express themselves in a way that reflects their personality. This can help women feel more empowered, positively impacting their mental and emotional well-being.

Embracing one's style during pregnancy can also help women remain connected to their sense of self. Pregnancy is a time of transformation; losing oneself amidst all the changes can be easy. However, by embracing their style, women can stay connected to their sense of self and authentically express themselves. This can help women feel more grounded and connected during significant change and transition.

DRESSING TIPS DURING THE DIFFERENT TRIMESTERS

FIRST TRIMESTER

During the first trimester of pregnancy, women may not yet have a visible bump, but their bodies undergo significant changes. Common symptoms like nausea, bloating, and fatigue can make it challenging to decide what to wear. However, with some creativity, it is still possible to look stylish and comfortable.

An excellent idea for a fashionable and comfortable outfit during the first trimester is to wear a flowy maxi dress with comfortable sandals. Maxi dresses are perfect for accommodating any bloating or changes in breast size during the first trimester. They are versatile and can be dressed up or down depending on the occasion. Pairing the dress with comfortable sandals will help keep your feet happy, especially if you are experiencing any swelling.

Another excellent option for a first-trimester outfit is to wear stretchy leggings or jeggings with a loose-fitting top. Look for tops made from breathable fabrics with a relaxed fit around the midsection to accommodate any bloating or changes in belly size. You can also accessorise this outfit with a statement necklace or scarf to draw attention away from any areas you may feel self-conscious.

Maternity jeans are another great option for the first trimester. They are designed to accommodate a growing belly and provide support where you need it most. You can pair them with a comfortable t-shirt or sweater for a casual look or dress them up with a blouse and blazer for a more formal occasion.

Lastly, comfortable shoes are essential during the first trimester. Your feet may start to swell, and you may experience some discomfort. Look for shoes that provide ample support and have a low or no heel. Flats, sneakers, and loafers are all great options that can be dressed up or down, depending on the outfit.

To sum up, choosing the right outfit during the first trimester can be challenging, but it is essential to prioritise comfort. Maxi dresses, leggings, maternity jeans, loose-fitting tops, and comfortable shoes are all great options. Remember to choose items that can accommodate changes in your body and reflect your style.

SECOND TRIMESTER

If you are in your second trimester of pregnancy, you may experience significant changes in your body. Finding comfortable and fashionable clothing can be challenging.

These tips will help you create a stylish outfit that accommodates your growing belly:

Start with a pair of comfortable, supportive maternity leggings or jeans. Look for those with a stretchy waistband that grows with you throughout your pregnancy. Pair them with a loose-fitting, flowy top that skims over your belly and provides plenty of room for movement. You can choose a solid colour or a fun, bold print to add personality to your outfit.

Add a lightweight cardigan or kimono to layer over your top. This will add warmth and dimension to your outfit. It can also help draw attention away from your growing belly and create a more balanced silhouette.

Choose comfortable, supportive footwear. Opt for low-heeled shoes or sneakers that provide good support and cushioning. Slip-on shoes or sandals with adjustable straps can be an excellent option for easy wear and adjustability as your feet may be swelling.

Accessorise with statement jewellery or a scarf. A bold necklace or earrings can draw attention to your face and create a focal point away from your belly. A scarf can add colour and texture to your outfit while providing warmth when needed.

Prioritise comfort and choose clothing that allows for movement and breathability. Do not be afraid to experiment with different styles and colours to find what works best for you. With these tips, you can create a fashionable and comfortable outfit that celebrates your growing belly and personal style.

THIRD TRIMESTER

As your pregnancy progresses into the third trimester, you may find it challenging to put together a stylish outfit due to the growing size of your belly. Do not worry, however! You can still look fashionable and feel confident with the following outfit ideas:

1. **Maxi Dress:** Opt for a maxi dress made of stretchable and breathable fabric to accommodate your growing belly. You can also accessorise with bold statement jewellery.

2. **Maternity Jeans and Flowy Top:** Maternity jeans are a must-have during pregnancy and can be styled in several ways. Pair them with a comfortable, airy top or blouse for that chic look. For footwear, flats or low-heeled booties can complete the outfit.

3. **Leggings and Tunic:** Leggings are a comfortable option that can be dressed up or down. Combine them with a long tunic or oversized sweater for a cosy and fashionable look. You can add ankle boots or sneakers to complete the outfit.

4. **Wrap Dress:** A wrap dress is a versatile piece that can

be dressed up or down. Make sure you choose a stretchy fabric that can accommodate your belly. Accessorise it with a belt to cinch in your waist and show off your bump.

5. **Jumpsuit:** A jumpsuit is a great option that can be stylish and comfortable. Select a jumpsuit with a stretchy waistband or a wrap-style top to accommodate your belly. Add statement earrings or a necklace for a more elegant look.

Remember, comfort, function, and style are the keys to feeling confident during the third trimester. Don't be afraid to experiment with different styles and accessories to find what works best for you.

With a little creativity, you can rock any outfit and feel beautiful throughout your pregnancy journey.

MIX AND MATCH DURING PREGNANCY

Mixing and matching outfits during pregnancy can be a fun and creative way to stay stylish and comfortable throughout your journey. With some knowledge and creativity, you can create a versatile wardrobe that can take you from day to night, work to play, and everything in between.

Here are some tips on how to mix and match outfits during pregnancy:

1. When creating your pregnancy wardrobe, it's best to begin with versatile basics that can be easily mixed and matched with other pieces. Opt for leggings, stretchy pants, basic tees, and tank tops. Seek out items made from stretchy and breathable fabrics that can adapt to your changing body throughout your pregnancy.

2. It is a great idea to invest in statement pieces for your wardrobe. These are the key items that add variety and interest to your look. They can include printed maxi dresses, patterned blouses, or statement jackets. Mix and match these pieces with your basics to create unique and stylish outfits. Having a few statement pieces in your wardrobe can elevate your style game and always look put together.

3. Layering is key: Layering is a great way to add depth and interest to your outfits while also providing versatility. Start with a basic tee or tank top and add layers such as a cardigan, blazer, or denim jacket. You can also layer dresses over leggings or wear a blouse over a dress for a unique and stylish look.

4. Don't be afraid to mix patterns: Mixing patterns can be a great way to add interest and variety to your outfits.

Start by choosing patterns that complement each other, such as stripes and florals or polka dots and checks. Keep the rest of your outfit simple and let the patterns be the focal point.

5. Use accessories to tie everything together: Accessories can be the final touch that ties your outfit together. This includes scarves, statement jewelry, belts, or hats. Focus on accessories that complement your outfit and add interest without overwhelming it.

6. Consider your lifestyle: When mixing and matching outfits, it's important to consider your lifestyle and the activities you'll be doing. You may need to focus on more professional looks if you work in an office. If you're a stay-at-home mom, you may want to focus on comfortable and casual outfits.

7. Don't forget about comfort: While style is important,

comfort is key during pregnancy. Choose clothing made from soft, stretchy fabrics that feel good against your skin. Make sure your shoes provide ample support and are comfortable to wear for long periods.

By following these tips, you can create a versatile and stylish wardrobe that will take you through your pregnancy journey confidently and comfortably. Remember to have fun and experiment with different looks to find what works best for you.

SELF-CARE

Taking care of one's mental health during pregnancy is crucial for both the mother and the child. Pregnancy is a time of significant change and can be stressful for many women. It is important to practice self-care during this time to ensure a healthy pregnancy and a healthy baby. This essay will discuss the importance of self-care and mental health during pregnancy.

Pregnancy can be a rollercoaster of emotions. Feeling anxious, stressed, and overwhelmed is normal during this time. However, it is essential to recognise when these feelings become too much to handle. Mental health issues such as depression and anxiety are common during pregnancy, and they can have severe consequences if left untreated. Studies have shown that untreated maternal depression can lead to preterm birth, low birth weight, and developmental delays in children.

Self-care is essential for maintaining good mental health during pregnancy. This includes getting enough rest, eating a healthy diet, and exercising regularly. Rest is crucial during pregnancy, as the body works hard to support the growing baby. It is essential to listen to your body and rest when necessary. Eating a healthy diet can help ensure both the mother and baby get the necessary nutrients. Exercise is also vital during pregnancy; it can help reduce stress and improve mood.

In addition to these basic self-care practices, there are many other things that women can do to take care of their mental health during pregnancy. One important step is to seek support from loved ones, friends, or a mental health professional. Talking about your feelings and concerns can help reduce stress and anxiety. Women should also try engaging in activities like reading, listening to music, or practising yoga.

Another important aspect of self-care during pregnancy is mindfulness. Mindfulness is the practice of being present at the moment and paying attention to your thoughts and feelings without judgment. It has been shown to reduce stress and improve mental health. There are many ways to practice mindfulness, such as meditation, deep breathing, or relaxing baths.

In conclusion, taking care of one's mental health during

pregnancy is essential for a healthy pregnancy and a healthy baby. Self-care practices such as getting enough rest, eating a healthy diet, and exercising regularly can help reduce stress and improve mood. Seeking support from loved ones or a mental health professional and engaging in activities that bring joy can also be helpful.

Finally, practising mindfulness can help reduce stress and improve mental health. Women can ensure a positive and healthy pregnancy experience by prioritising self-care and mental health during pregnancy.

CONCLUSION

In this book, we have delved into the various stages of pregnancy and the ways in which your body transforms during each trimester. We have also discussed the types of clothing that are best suited for each stage, how to mix and match different pieces to create stylish outfits, and how to accessorize during pregnancy. Nonetheless, this book is not solely about fashion, but also about accepting your changing body and relishing the journey of pregnancy.

During pregnancy, it's crucial to prioritize your comfort. Your body is undergoing incredible changes and needs the necessary care and support. Choose clothes that accommodate your growing belly and offer support where you need it the most. Maternity wear is specifically designed to meet these needs, so don't hesitate to invest in a few essential pieces that will help you feel comfortable and confident throughout your pregnancy.

Embracing your pregnancy style is not just about dressing up. It also involves taking care of your mental and emotional well-being. Pregnancy can bring a lot of emotional changes, and it is crucial to prioritize your mental and emotional health during this time. You can achieve this by doing activities like prenatal yoga, meditation, or just by taking some time out for yourself. Remember to make your mental and emotional well-being a priority throughout your pregnancy.

During pregnancy, it's important to not shy away from experimenting with your style. Try out various colors, patterns, and textures to find what makes you feel good about yourself and enhances your beauty. You can add some personality to your outfits by accessorizing them with statement jewelry, scarves or hats. Keep in mind, pregnancy is a phase of changes and growth, and your fashion choices can reflect that.

Looking great during pregnancy is more than just a matter of appearance. It involves accepting the changes that come with pregnancy, prioritizing comfort and mental well-being, and enjoying the experience. Whether you're expecting for the first time or have been through it before, this book provides you with the knowledge and creativity to look and feel your best throughout your pregnancy. So embrace your pregnancy style, have fun with your fashion choices, and enjoy this beautiful journey with confidence and grace.

**Congratulations and best wishes on embarking
on your journey to motherhood!**

ABOUT THE AUTHOR

Sharon Shante

Sharon Shante, a mother of three, has always been passionate about elegance and class. She believes that women face challenges in breaking stereotypes and pushing boundaries. Through her book, she hopes to guide and inspire women to become sophisticated and graceful. Sharon's journey towards elegance and class is proof that it's not just about appearance or attire, but also about how you carry yourself, how you treat others, and how you make an impact in the world.

BOOKS BY THIS AUTHOR

The Elegant And Classy Woman

In today's fast-paced, modern world, elegance and class can sometimes feel like a thing of the past. However, the truth is that these qualities are more critical than ever before. At a time when social media and popular culture often promote superficiality and materialism, it is essential to remember the value of inner beauty, confidence, and grace.

This book guides women who want to cultivate elegance and class. It is not about being perfect or following strict rules but about embracing your unique qualities and radiating positivity and confidence in everything you do.

Radiate Confidence And Poise

The book "Radiate Confidence and Poise: A Woman's Guide to Unleashing Inner Strength and Grace" is a comprehensive guide that helps women develop the essential confidence and poise necessary to succeed in all aspects of life. It is based on extensive research, personal experiences, expert insights, communication, and personal development.